# The Inner Darkness

'My Own True Story'

# Gladys Medcroft

**chipmunkapublishing**
the mental health publisher

Published by
Chipmunkapublishing
United Kingdom

**http://www.chipmunkapublishing.com**

ISBN    978-1-78382-234-8

## About The Author

If you saw Gladys going about her daily business you would not look twice. Just another housewife, a mother, one who gets on with the chores of life.

It is not everyone though who has enough courage to tell of deeply personal trials and tragedies. Not a story told to seek praise, but in the hope that it may help others to understand.

This book only touches on her dedication to helping others. She is a true friend to those she continues to visit in hospital or call on at home in their time of need. She makes no mention of the years she has devoted to The Southmead User Network. Hers is not a passive role, she has always pushed to make life better for others.

Whether a major event, or a weekly or monthly meeting, Gladys is always to be found at the forefront of the action.

**Chapter 1**

Much of my early life is now a blurred memory, but I still recollect the cold, the hunger and the constant moving from place to place as we sought for somewhere to live.

I was born in Totnes but shortly afterwards we all moved to London – my parents, sisters' brother and myself. We were living in squalid conditions in ex-army huts without furniture, but with blankets to keep us warm. As the huts became due for demolition, so our few possessions were loaded on to an old pram and we set out to try to find another. I can remember being woken by an official of some sort shining a torch on us and saying that we would have to go as the hut was due to come down.

At one time things became so bad that we literally had nowhere to sleep and we all went into a prison for the night.

Travelling around trying to find somewhere to live we eventually arrived in Bristol where we lived for a while in an ex-army hut, which was built on stilts.

My father had a drink problem and when the worse for drink he couldn't negotiate the steps up to the hut and frequently ended up underneath it. Although as a father he was inadequate, he did his best.

As far as I remember we always had food and blankets to keep us warm at night. However, when we had to leave our latest 'home' there was nowhere else for us to go but the workhouse in Fishponds Road.

We children were split up and I went first to Vinney Green Children's Home, and at a later date was transferred to Downend Homes, as were the other children. I felt like a pawn continuously moved around.

We were all in No. 2 house. Years went by, my elder sister left and we were all separated and moved into different houses, which really upset us. Every time I was missing I was in the nursery. I loved that. I had a brother and sister there. They were later fostered.

There was very strict discipline. At 6.00 a.m. we were lined up and given our duties – bedmaking, peeling potatoes, mending and so on.

There were so many different things to be done. Before we went to school we were again lined up like an army. A button missing or a hole in a sock meant we were sent for after school and reprimanded. Every Saturday we were given sixpence to spend in the tuck shop, but any misdemeanour meant we didn't get our pocket money.

They looked after us well but it was nothing like a real home; love there was none, and without that life for a child is empty.

While at Downend we attended church regularly and as I became older I was given charge of the young ones on Sundays. The staff never discovered that I often took them to a different church where I fancied a boy in the choir, who used to sometimes come to the home for functions like sports day. I enjoyed out-witting the staff and the little ones never told.

Later I became very involved at our recognised church, which I then attended regularly and I asked to be confirmed. As the classes had already started, I took them on my own.

The day of confirmation arrived and I was very annoyed. It was a solemn occasion – we were all in white and the church was very quiet. Suddenly my mother and father who had come for the ceremony were fighting and arguing in the church. It spoilt my day. My father had bought me a skirt, but although I should have liked to have it, I wouldn't. I didn't know where he got it from, he could have come by it honestly, but I couldn't be sure.

Often at holiday times, and sometimes weekends, people would arrive whom we called aunties or uncles. They sometimes brought presents and sometimes took us out to tea or home for the weekend. No doubt their intentions were good and they were kind to us, but for me it was never a success. Where they had children of their own I found it impossible to mix.

I felt so ill at ease and unsure of how I should behave with the result that I was very silent. I dare say they thought I was sullen and ungrateful, but they couldn't understand how I felt.

## Chapter 2

When I was about fourteen I went to a foster home, where I was very happy with my own little room, and I could watch television. I had now started working. My first job was at a drinking straw factory, which I didn't like very much but stuck at it because I was secure and contented. Unfortunately my foster parents were getting elderly and decided they didn't want the responsibility, so I had to move to a hostel. Although I knew it couldn't continue I was very sad as they had been kind and understood children, as they had brought up a large family. I kept in touch with them and used to go back to see them on Sundays after church and have dinner and tea with them. Margaret – my foster sister – came too. After tea I went back to the hostel and so to bed. Each morning I got up – prepared my breakfast, usually cereal and toast, then off to catch my bus. The matron, when I was first at the hostel, was Mrs Munroe.

The money we earned we gave to her; so much she kept for board, some she saved for us for clothes and the rest she gave back as pocket money for make-up, toilet goods and the like.

I shared a bedroom with a nice girl called Anne – we got on well. It was a pleasant place and we had plenty of freedom to come and go. There were four bedrooms on the top floor, bathroom and toilet. One floor down was the staff room and another bedroom with bathroom and toilet.

Next going down was the big dayroom with armchairs and television. Also on this floor was the assistant matron's room and her office. The basement floor comprised the dining room and kitchen, storeroom and laundry. Our evening and Sunday meals were taken in a separate room where there were four dining tables. If any of us were out of work we helped out with the meals, and those home earliest from work also gave a hand. After a while, Mrs Munroe left and Mrs Worgan took over. Miss Daw, or Marge, as we called her was assistant matron.

Mrs Haines came in daily to help with the cooking. Miss Burgess, a dear old soul, used to do the cleaning – she brought her little dog with her.

As soon as I was working I tried to help my mother and father as much as possible, although I did not have much money myself. At this time they were living in two rooms in Bath. My father could not or would not get a job and they were constantly short of money. Most Saturdays I would go over on the bus, then to the food shops to buy what I could afford before visiting them.

The one thing my father could find money for was face powder, which he made my mother use to cover up the bruises he inflicted. I should have preferred just to give to my mother, but I knew it would cause rows if I did that.

In the hostel we had a record player. They gave me a record of Elvis Presley's 'Wooden Heart' and I was always playing it, much to the annoyance of the other girls.

I used to go to the Glen dancing and on one occasion a girl stepped on my toe and I had a bad foot. I wouldn't get any treatment but finally I was forced to as it became poisoned. I had to have my nail off at the hospital and stay home from work, as I couldn't stand on my foot, and bathe it every day in very hot, salt water.

Wednesdays we all went to a club and while my foot was bad my friends carried me up the stairs. We had some interesting speakers to teach us various things, which we had never had any opportunity to learn about like dress sense and make-up. At one time, Shirley Bassey's make-up girl came.

I left the straw factory because the journey was too long and had a succession of miscellaneous jobs. After a couple of weeks without a job, the Labour Exchange sent me to a transport café. I enjoyed it there – I liked meeting the customers, but I found money confusing and usually ended up charging less than I should.

I could see it wouldn't be long before the manageress asked me to go, so I forestalled her by leaving there. In those days it was quite easy to get work provided one was flexible and didn't mind having a try at various things.

I enjoyed my next job, which was in a paint factory where the work was rotated so it didn't become too tedious. Sometimes I was filling the tins, sometimes stamping the colour on the top, or maybe stacking or other work.

While I was at the paint factory I made a good friend, Maureen. Four of us, Maureen and Bob who were later married, myself and Bill, went everywhere together.

I was engaged to Bill for a year but decided I didn't want to marry him. Unfortunately, from the day I started there was one woman in the same team as myself who was continually harassing and criticising me. Now, I would not let myself get upset by such a person, but then I was young and vulnerable. One day when she had been particularly vindictive, I could stand it no longer. I had a tin of paint in my hand and I poured it over her head. That, of course, was marching orders for me.

So long as I was working, the hostel staff didn't concern themselves with where I was, so when I left the factory I went straight into the Co-op Laundry and asked if they had a job for me. There was a vacancy so I started there right away. Here again, I had various duties – sorting the laundry; pressing the sheets on large rollers; filling the dryers, etc. After a few months I left, as I found work at a printing firm, which was not such a long journey for me. I couldn't settle for very long anywhere so I changed again and had a spell at a Corporation Department serving dinners, and clearing tables.

## Chapter 3

I decided to have a change and took a post in an old people's home. I loved the old people but the work was sheer slavery. On one occasion the husband and wife went away leaving myself (I was about eighteen then) and another girl (slightly older) to look after the old people. After they had gone we found the only food they had left was biscuits and cheese, so that day we could only give them that for their tea. The next day we had to buy food from our own money to feed them.

Much as I loved the old people I couldn't stand the drudgery and so I left. I was by this time finding the home life too restrictive and thought it was time I stood on my own feet, so I found a residential post at the BRI. There I lived in the maids' hostel.

I cleaned the nurses' bedrooms, also the sisters' bedrooms, which were in another block. I took them tea and breakfast in bed. Sometimes I also helped on relief in the matron's house. I still go back to see the ladies – it was a smashing place.

The painters came in to paint the nurses' home, among them being a fellow called Ron. Although I was still going out with Bill, I started seeing Ron and at weekends we went out all the time. Often we went to Dursley and stayed the night with Ron's brother, Bill, and his wife Rosalyn. Ron could get all the work he wanted in the building trade, so we were able to go out and enjoy ourselves when we wanted to.

While I was at the BRI the Sister of the Nurses' Home found out my reading and writing problem, also the fact that I had never had the opportunity to learn to cook or tackle things alone. This was worrying me as I hoped to get married. She was very helpful and arranged for me to learn something about cooking in the O. T. Department every Wednesday afternoon.

Then on a Thursday afternoon I went to the Army School at Corsham where they had a class for soldiers with reading problems. It was interesting but I think I learned more about guns, under-carriages, etc., than I did about reading.

When I was about twenty, Ron and I became engaged and we married the following year.

We had to wait until then, as my father wouldn't give his consent – he had no reason for his refusal, it was part of his vindictive nature.

We found a flat in Cotham and I moved in two weeks before the wedding to get it all ready. It was the middle flat with the living room one side and the bedroom the other. The bathroom was on the next floor up and we shared it with the family there. The flat was in a terrible condition but Ron was able to decorate.

I was married at St. Michael's church. I had three bridesmaids, two in yellow and one in blue. The material was satin and they wore white shoes and a flower in their hair. We gave them Prayer books as a present, which they carried with them.

I wore a long, full white satin wedding dress with layers of lace on top, a matching headdress and a floral cross of roses. We had a lovely reception, which would not have been possible if the BRI had not helped out with the

catering. My Uncle Fred made the wedding cake as a present as that was his profession.

I left the BRI as obviously I didn't want a residential post and went to work at Bolloms in the canteen, preparing dinners and teas for the workers in the factory.

We were eager to start a family and after about seven months I was pleased to leave as by then I was expecting a baby. In due course I had a baby boy, Brian, who was born in the Bristol Maternity Hospital. We were happy all the time we were married. We lived in Cotham for three years, then moved to a council flat at Withywood. Two years after Brian was born I had a miscarriage, but later I had a little girl, Linda.

Life went on day after day, month after month. Going to the shops, looking after the babies, taking them when older to school, preparing meals for Ron.

We discovered that my father had cancer and he died quite soon afterwards. A few years later my mother developed cancer of the lung. We went to visit her at home as often as possible, first at the women's hostel and later a council flat until she died from the disease.

When I was a little girl I missed much of my schooling in the early days, so I had a speech problem including a very severe stutter.

Years after, the doctor put me in touch with a speech therapist at Clifton, and my speech problem was overcome. But I was still left with reading and writing difficulties.

As a result of this I had a very unpleasant experience in a Bank where I was accused of forgery. Needless to say, I have never been back to that Bank. I learned to cope in various ways, not always very successfully, as I would, for example, arrive home with a birthday card with completely unsuitable words.

Ron woke up one morning and said, "I am going to the doctor, I've a lump on my neck which I think is a carbuncle." The doctor sent him to the hospital for tests and he was later admitted - neither of us realised how serious his condition was or what his prospects were likely to be. The doctor took me aside and told me he had Hodgkin's disease, which I had never heard of, and that his future was bleak and limited.

I shut my mind to what he was saying. I was not in the room, I was at school, at home, anywhere but where my body was. His words meant nothing to me at the time.

I was told later that he would live anything between six months and fifteen years. The doctor asked me if he should be told, but I said, "No, I will tell him when the right moment comes."

In the event he lived for three years, in and out of hospital for treatment but he didn't know until the last six months the truth regarding his condition, neither did he know that I knew all along.

So the nightmare began as his condition deteriorated and the treatment he was receiving produced horrific side effects. Still not aware of how desperately ill he was, he was trying determinedly to lead a normal life not realising that this was impossible. Each day brought its own problems and fears.

Whenever we went out in the car I wondered if disaster was ahead. Hanging on to the seat, shouting at the children and watching him for any signs of collapse, which happened periodically and involved various parts of the body – eyes, hands and feet. Each journey seemed an endless hell. Continually watching his speed, shouting at him to go slower if he exceeded thirty miles per hour, him shouting back at me not realising why I was so scared, built up severe tension between us and the children.

He was on a limited diet, certain foodstuffs being forbidden. Without realising he was doing it he became very difficult to cater for. For instance, I well remember the day when he said he would like fish. I started cooking it and suddenly he said, "I don't want fish, I would like liver." Episodes like this happened repeatedly.

Looking back I realise that it was the effect of the illness or the treatment. At the time I couldn't see this, and suffered further strain and tension. What a contrast from earlier years when he was fit and well. Then, as Sunday was my day off Ron cooked my breakfast for me; off I went with the children while he prepared dinner, afterwards cleaning up before taking us off to Weston or family visiting.

Now he started to have blackouts and the situation was similar to the experiences in the car. As I lifted him up, he usually came round and demanded to know what I was doing, having no recollection of having fallen, and again we ended up shouting at each other. Bath time was another horror. Always he liked a lot of water, and I tried desperately to persuade him to have less. Terrified that he might have a blackout while in the water I dare not move far from the bathroom, to prevent him from suspecting I was hovering near, to rush in if needed. I had to help him in and out of the bath, which he much resented, and each time he had a course of treatment Ron became progressively worse.

When he realised the gravity of his illness his attitude changed.

Nothing was said between us but he started buying more things for the house such as a washing machine to make things easier for me. He was also telling me not to hit the children and to look after them, and if I wanted to get married again I should do so. I made no reply, but I knew from his remarks that he was aware that he wouldn't be here long.

So the time went on until a day came when Ron drove to the hospital and was admitted immediately. Obviously he should not have been driving, but he was so independent that he refused an ambulance as he had on other occasions, and his willpower gave him strength to get there. I was with him and stayed with him settling him in. Now, for roughly a month my life revolved between home, hospital and school. In the evenings it meant taking the children to the hospital; they spent many hours in the library or corridors.

The day came when I took the children to see their father for what I knew would be the last time. The following night he was in a one-bed cubicle.

I sat for many hours by his bed, I must have fallen asleep and when I came round I was lying on a bed.

I went back in and stayed with him until he died the following afternoon. My first feelings were of intense relief for the children and myself. I felt in a whirl and didn't know what to do. After the intense activity of the last few weeks I had come to a full stop.

My mother-in-law had come to stay, and Uncle Ted made the funeral arrangements. Flowers were sent to the house, which was full of relations who took charge of proceedings. I felt completely detached from it all and was thinking about other things. The day after the funeral my mother-in-law went home and I was left alone with the children.

Gladys Medcroft

## Chapter 4

About a week later I developed signs of hyperactivity, which alternated with periods of complete inactivity. I spent hours watching television, identifying the characters with relations, but the bad characters I obsessively identified with myself. Another symptom was that I sat for hours watching the clock on the stove looking for consolation.

I developed a terror of people and thought they were following me. Cars also frightened me, every driver had Ron's face, but I couldn't stop myself looking in them. I had a feeling of being closed in but was scared to go out.

I avoided all people but men in particular terrified me, even to the point that I thought they were trying to photograph me in my bath and all the time the light bulbs were flashing. I thought I was being watched and

photographed all the time. Sometimes I had spells of intense activity and danced wildly until exhausted before slumping into a chair and falling asleep.

I disowned my name and my ring. I still tried to go to work, but sometimes I couldn't bear the place or the people, although they really tried to help me. On one occasion I wrote a letter and gave it to a man at work, although I hadn't written it for him but for another dear friend; this particular workmate never knew how he helped me just by talking to me.

I said many things, which were true to me in my fantasy world, but had no real truth in them.

Sometimes between whiles I realised what I had been saying but could find no way to rectify it. I felt guilty and stupid and stayed away from work more and more.

The money from the Insurance cane through and I spent wildly but not without purpose. I replaced a lot of furniture – I didn't want any remainders of the past. I started taking the children out, using taxis in which I felt safe. I had to make myself shop for food otherwise the children would have gone hungry. The money was no object. I did not consider it was mine and was trying to get rid of it. We went on holidays, had meals out and generally spent the money until it was gone.

By now I was doing a lot of walking, but I was always looking for somewhere safe. A day came when I felt desperate. I went to the local churches – if they had been open - if I could have found someone to answer my cry for help, what happened next would never have come about.

I walked all the way to the centre of the city, several miles in a daze, and found myself eventually in the Lord Mayor's Chapel, an historic building in Bristol. Once there, I sat down and started to cry. I couldn't stop and I cried for three hours, hiding my face. There was a member of the chapel staff there, who tried to help me in my distress, but I couldn't express what was happening. Eventually he had to send for the police – he had no choice – but I thought he was against me, and I couldn't understand what I had done wrong. Once in the police care I felt relaxed and safe and was able to talk coherently.

They gave me a cup of tea and I waited until eventually a welfare officer arrived at Bridewell and took me home.

In my desperation I had started drinking, any time, day or night. I was drinking sherry and even took it to work with me concealed in a container.

The doctor came to see me and prescribed tablets but I did not take them. I had enough sense to realise the danger involved in taking them while drinking heavily. A day came when I bought a bottle of whisky, took it home and drank nearly the whole bottle. I can recollect gathering up the children's clothes and throwing them all out of the window. Neighbours thought I had taken an overdose and called an ambulance, and I was taken to Southmead Hospital. When I was on the bed I heard someone say, "She's drunk."

I was calling the name of a gentleman who had been very kind and helpful to me, but in my confused state I thought the doctor was this man. After a while I came home and cleared up all the mess I had made, the children staying with a neighbour for the night.

The following day relatives arrived who had been contacted by my neighbour. I kept the doors locked and took no notice of their pleading to be let in. I was watching the clock; there was only one person I felt I could trust and he would arrive home at six o'clock. When he got home I asked for him to come in, but nobody else. I didn't want them and at my request he told them to go away, which they did. We talked for a long time and I felt calmer and more relaxed.

Things continued about the same; flashing lights, compulsive washing, fear of people in general and suspicion of neighbours. I had a strange experience when I went through all the motions of a pregnancy, continuing for nine months.

My periods stopped my stomach and breasts enlarged and I felt movements as of a baby kicking. Although I knew a pregnancy was impossibility at the time, I didn't accept this and was quite pleased to think I was having a baby, and told people it would be arriving at any time. Some time later, it all just drifted away and was forgotten.

On several occasions I made my son ring for the police who came to reassure me and calm me down. Fear of going out continued. I couldn't bear to see his – my husband's –face revealed on the features of every man I passed.

One day I went on one of my long walks and went into a church at Fishponds. At first I just sat and looked at the altar, then, suddenly, I felt everything was wrong. The Bible was open on the lectern so I changed the page, also opened the hymnbooks in the pews. Why? I don't know. I meant no harm. I left an offering in the box on the wall.

When I was in the house I would sometimes be impelled to gather up lots of bits and pieces, put them on the bed and try to make a crucifix from them. It was like a puzzle as seen before but not remembered. I had to try and put it together. I wouldn't let anyone else see it.

## Chapter 5

Finally things reached a climax. It must have been early morning with just enough light to see what I was doing.

In the garden I lit a fire. I piled things on – all the things, which had belonged to Ron, - anything he had touched. It wasn't me, it was if another personality had taken over, yet I was still in sufficient control not to destroy furniture or anything like that. Then I started washing, gathering up clothes etc., and bundling them into the machine. This half done I suddenly went upstairs and said to the children, "Quick, get up, we must get out."

I wrapped blankets around them and went out. I felt desperate to find a house showing a light. When I did, I rang the bell and a lady came to the door, took us in, and made me a cup of tea. In the meantime her husband fetched the police. I wanted to go home, but they took the children from me and took us, separately, to the police station. Then a policeman took the children home after asking if there was anyone who would look after them. I told them my sister and sister-in-law's address. I was really frightened.

Someone who said he was a doctor told me to sign a form, which I did. I didn't know what I was signing, but I was consenting to be admitted to Glenside.

They wanted me to go straight there but I insisted on going home first. I said the house was dirty and the fire might be still burning. When we arrived it was just smouldering and the house was, of course, perfectly clean.

They took me back to the station and I heard them say, "She'll go to Glenside." I didn't want to go and struggled with them but of course, it was no good.

An ambulance came and picked me up, I heard them say, "she'll be trouble," but when we arrived there I got out and went quietly to Mason Unit. I felt safe and a great relief. I was resentful and didn't want to do as I was told, or take the tablets prescribed. For the first few days I was not allowed out, but later, provided I asked for permission, I could, and I went for long walks. I was still suffering from 'visions' and confusions. I was running away wanting to go home, but also to go back, although actually, I was over the worst before I went in. I stayed three weeks. My escape from reality to relieve tension was through music and dancing.

Although I still, off and on, sat for periods in a state of withdrawal, at the same time I knew almost immediately I wanted to help the others. One patient who was always wetting the bed would not do anything she was told, wouldn't go for breakfast – she came for me.

Another time a patient smashed a window. I stayed with her although the other patients said she was violent. I picked up the glass and consoled her.

An old lady of dirty habits I took under my wing, put her in the bath, washed her and her clothes. I just had to help these people; others couldn't seem to reach them.

When the children came to see me, I knew deep down they were mine, but didn't feel as if they belonged to me.

However, I tore the 'No Admittance' notices from the doors of the rooms where visitors were not allowed, and took them in. I was never stopped, although the notices were replaced. I don't like regulations.

One night I was restless and went for a walk out of the ward. I went through the unit to a room where repairs were being done. Paper was smouldering. I stamped it out and just then a staff member came in and said, "What are you doing there?" I ran back to bed. I didn't tell anyone – who would have believed me?

When I went in I only had the clothes I was wearing. I wanted to wash them, so out of the nightdress provided, I made a garment of sorts to wear while my other clothes dried, or someone brought me some more in. The staff did not comment directly, but I felt they thought it was part of my condition, which made me do it. It wasn't, I just wanted something to wear.

I still wanted to be a different person, influenced, I think, by television. I pulled down the curtains in the bedroom and made myself a sari. How, I don't know, or why. Shortly afterwards my brain clicked back, how else can I describe it, and I realised what I had done.

Two of my relations came in and told me a relation had died. I was in the kitchen at the time and they came in and said they had something to tell me. They didn't need to say anything, I knew, as they were wearing black ties. The other relatives didn't think I should be told, they thought I would be upset. Why? Why are people afraid of dying?

After a few days I was allowed to go down to the shops on my own.

What a relief! Before that if I wanted to go out it was only possible if someone was available to go with me. It was so humiliating. When I was allowed home for a weekend I felt as if I was being released from prison. It seemed as if I was there a long time, every day was a year. I wanted to get home to see a special friend. Actually, I was only there for three weeks.

I felt I had to be working all the time. I laid up the trolley at night and cleaned the kitchen. We were supposed to take turns at preparing things in the morning, but I always got them ready the night before. I had to keep on the go. I couldn't sit and watch TV for long. I found it too frightening.

In the mornings there was group therapy – how I detested it. We sat round in a circle and had to repeat our names. When it came to me I walked out and wouldn't go back. They treated us like children, it was supposed to be voluntary, but we were expected to attend. The theory was that we should practice free expression, and it was supposed to help by releasing tension. It never did anything for me. I felt the whole procedure to be childish and ridiculous. I found more help by talking individually to other patients, their problems – not mine.

Alternatively, I turned to music. Drug therapy I didn't want. Whatever the tablets were that I was given, they didn't help. I am not speaking for others, maybe they cannot help themselves, and need firm guidance and therapy. I did my best to help some of them. Often in the beginning they were abusive, but I took no notice. Later they came to me. It is no good dwelling on your own problems – we were all there for the same reasons.

I think the major deficiency is that there is nowhere for patients to give vent to their feelings. Most of the patients can feel when unbearable tension is arising within them, which they must release. A small, soundproof cubicle where one could scream or otherwise react, would save such a lot of embarrassment and possibly avoid harm both to the patient and the others in the ward.

The other service, which is very badly needed, is for someone to be available when wanted someone apart from the Psychiatrist who is always busy. Not just at set times, but to be there when wanted. It is not necessary for that person to be a doctor, who anyway has a frightening effect on the patients. A person who is not afraid to handle violence and can understand the needs of the patient. It is the most un-cooperative who needs the most help.

Many of the patients were afraid to go downstairs after tea, to the phone or for any other reason. I wasn't worried about it at all, and would go down with them. I treated them as if they were normal people and tried to encourage them to talk to me.

There was one person of the staff who was really great. I called her the Sergeant Major. She was apparently as hard as nails – no nonsense from anybody, but a real softie underneath. She had a way with her and could get round you without realising it.

After about three weeks, which seemed like forever, they said I looked a lot better and would I like to go home, so I went. The children came home. It felt very strange and I wanted to tell them to go away. I didn't feel it was time to see them. This was a first reaction, which only lasted a couple of days.

**Chapter 6**

My neighbours, an old lady and her son, were very helpful over this period, but kept giving me soup, which I did not want. I became very friendly with them and they sustained me over a difficult period.

They had asked me at the hospital if I worked and advised me not to go back for a while.

However, I went straight back, although I dreaded going because of all the things I had said and done. In the event, although naturally they seemed a bit apprehensive about how I might behave, they treated me just the same. I had to get a doctor's note to allow me to return and then everything was as it had been before.

I still had some problems, but these were largely due to a private problem of a personal nature. I could not watch on television any programme, which I could identify with my own experience.

This continued for quite a long time but had I not had the breakdown I could have coped more readily with my current difficulties. Although I had theoretically recovered from my breakdown, I was still suffering the effects. I do not think the authorities realise how long the effects last.

My experience had made me very interested in mental illness and the way it affected people and the way authorities resolve their treatment.

I was by then attending a Group Therapy meeting and I became involved with other people and their reactions.

Also, I wanted to recall how I felt when I was under the influence of drink. I started drinking sherry, but I tried to stand outside of myself, and watch my own and other people's reactions. This was very difficult, and eventually I found it was getting out of my control, and I had to ask for help. I received the help and through this I learned more, because I could analyse the doctor's reaction.

I started taping my experience, but I found emotional complications so had to abandon it. I asked if I might sit in another group of more afflicted persons. I felt I wanted to learn more of other peoples' feelings and their problems. This did not come about, but our own group, by general agreement, became self-sufficient.

As new arrivals came, I would directly approach them and try to reassure them. (If they needed it there was always professional help available). Naturally there was great variation in their behaviour – some very talkative, some very silent, others very tearful, but this would occur in any group of people.

I noticed that as improvement was made and confidence returned, people could help others, often without realising they were doing so.

Whilst I was going to Group at Southmead, one of the staff of whom I enquired about voluntary work at Glenside, put me in touch with Mrs Cox and an appointment was made with her. There I became very anxious as to whether I ought to tell her I had had a breakdown, so I asked my doctor who said there was no need.

It took several days to catch him as I waited outside the surgery to see him, as he didn't attend every day. I was so needlessly worried as to what they would ask me.

When I arrived Mrs Cox made me feel very much at home, so much so that after a few minutes I told her I had been a patient there. She took me up to a ward and introduced me to a patient – Flo – and also the staff. I went two afternoons a week and took bits and pieces such as knitting squares, unravelling tangled embroidery threads, puzzle books, crayons and crayoning books.

I tried to get them all interested in something. Flo was my particular friend. I took her to town and also brought her home with me. We went to the Wild Life Park where she really enjoyed feeding the animals. After we got back home she started to get restless, she knew her meal was at six o'clock and she would rather get back than have a meal with me. She worried about her duties and the routine things she usually did.

Only once did I have difficulty with her. We went locally for a walk and sat on a log. Suddenly she developed a frightening tantrum. I had great difficulty in getting her back, but once well away from the spot she was all right. I didn't take her that way again. Was it some past memory?

Time went on and sometimes I had a little group to talk to. I also went on another ward to see Mary whom I had known before. She recognised me, although I hadn't seen her for many years. She had nobody who cared.

If more people visited they would have a truer idea of the patients concerned and might lose some of the false impressions they have.

The tension and strain continued to build up, and eventually the doctor said he thought it would be a good idea if I went into Glenside. He sent me home to pack my case, which actually I had already done. I could tell I needed hospital help. He took me to the hospital himself and made sure I was on the same ward as I had been in previously. By the time I was admitted I was really over the worst of the illness. It appears to me that action is usually delayed too long and a lot of hardship could be prevented with earlier diagnosis and assistance.

I adapted very quickly and assisted on the ward. Once I was in there I felt secure and my worries disappeared; I think because I only had myself to look after. At the same time I was still thinking about home, and when I had been in there three weeks I was urging them to discharge me. I said I had to go to the Bank and pay the coalman, so they let me go out and spend one night at home. On my return next day they said I could be discharged.

I suppose they might have been trying me out the day before to see what would happen.

It felt strange at first, I missed the company and I returned to work as soon as I possibly could. I needed to get out of the house and re-adjust to my normal routine. I was on quite high medication, but fortunately, now I have been able to reduce them considerably. For the first time in my life, I feel I am 'me' a real person adequately equipped to deal with anything life may present.

I now try to help others who may have similar problems, and also visit hospital patients who, for one reason or another, have no visitors.

When in a depression one is liable to say or do things, which you don't mean at all, but can really hurt someone and drive them away. If people could ignore it, sit and say nothing, which I know is very hard, they would do a great service. The outburst is beyond control and afterwards you want to say, "I didn't do or say it", but of course you did.

It is very difficult afterwards to overcome the effects of an antagonism aroused in this way. If only people would accept that it is all part of the illness. It is as though for a short time another personality dominates you, taking over control. This may only last a few minutes, but it may be hours or even days. This is not the real 'you'. It is a terrifying experience – you wonder if you will ever recover your normality.

I shall always be grateful to the people I work with for helping my recovery, even though they may not be aware that they did.

## Chapter 7

The right sort of help goes a long way towards shortening the duration of the illness. During the recovery period, which is in some ways the most difficult time, one is aware that people are watching, nervously waiting for some abnormal speech or behaviour. This only increases the strain and tension and makes recovery more difficult, as one is then hypersensitive about what people will say to them. A friendly approach and natural conversation does much to assist the person on the road back to normality.

A tape recording:

This is Gladys Medcroft,

Hello,

I am trying to do a survey on people with a mental health problem. Well, I hope I am going to say it clear and correct.

When I was in Glenside a long time ago, I was trying to do a little bit of research myself although I was ill. Anyway, I found when people were ill and they had done something unusual, probably in the hospital or outside the hospital; when the police, social workers, doctor or nurses, or whoever was involved, asked the patient why they had done what they'd done, they would probably get some abuse. Because the patient cannot understand why they had done such a thing.

If that person was left for half an hour or so to sit quietly and think of what they had done, they would probably feel quite silly and embarrassed and would, by then, be much more co-operative. However, it would depend on how deep their depression is.

If they are very, very depressed they could do things such as smashing a window or hit out at somebody quite violently. But if they were not in a deep depression they might just go into a room in the hospital, like I did, and take a pair of tights or something similar. They might go into a church and change things around, like I did when I walked all the way to Fishponds. Some people do much worse things and the police become involved, with the result that the person just feels silly and very embarrassed. The police then call a psychiatrist or doctor, but sometimes the patient doesn't want to say why they have done anything silly or dangerous, to them they have just been hitting out at something. Something in the brain has prompted them to do so and they are unable to resist whatever it is that trips them off.

As I have said before, if they were left for an hour when they were like this, then whoever is dealing with them could go back and ask again if the person wishes to tell them anything. At the time they probably feel very embarrassed to tell anyone about things. What I am trying to find out is what does happen when a patient is like this.

All I know at the moment is that they are very highly strung and they are trying to tell somebody something, but are unable to explain what it is they want to say.

I used to do a lot of dancing and I was trying to push, push it out of my mind and get on with something else.

Often I would lock myself away in a bedroom as long as possible, until I realised I had come back to normal, but a lot of people do not realise this and they stay out in the open. I am talking about a hospital now, where people are sitting out in the open and not in a room of their own. Why couldn't there be a room in Glenside, for instance, where patients could just let themselves go, like a rubber room. They have these in some children's places, not a children's hospital but in homes for handicapped children. The children can go into these rooms and throw themselves about, punch things, etc. There's nothing in the room that would allow them to hurt themselves.

I am more than sure that this would help. I hope I am trying to put it over quite clearly to you. If the patient could go to a room like this when they have a bout of depression where they could scream and shout and punch, I know this would help. I think this would help to get a lot of things out of their system instead of being prescribed more drugs. This is what the patient needs at that time, not more drugs. At a time like this they can be very rude and abusive and generally be in a right 'pickle'. Doctors then say that they have a very difficult patient.

The patient will then go very quiet and won't tell you anything and become generally withdrawn. Obviously they get very embarrassed.

## Chapter 8

When I was at work a long time ago (I've worked in the same place for a long time), we were talking about going on holiday, and someone said something about swimming costumes. I said that I would show them my costume, and the next day I went into work, went into the ladies toilet, put on my swimming costume and paraded up and down in front of everyone.

Normally, I would never have dreamt of doing this. I am just trying to give an example of a funny incident, but also there could be a dangerous situation like juggling with the traffic. The traffic is coming at you from all sides; people are swearing at you and telling you to get out of the way. Next thing they get the law out, drag you down to the police station, and by the time you get down there you're feeling all right and just want to go home. Realising your predicament you get into a right state.

An example is I woke up one night at 3 o'clock in the morning. You don't see many lights, but any lights that were on were a friend, everyone else was an enemy. I went to this lady's house with my children.

I wouldn't leave my children alone in the house, they were too young then. The man of the house went to the police, the police came and dragged me into a car, then took my children away from me. I was screaming and shouting, I was partly mental and partly sane. I wanted my children; I wondered where they were taking me. I was taken to the police station. After a while a man came, a doctor from the clinic.

I was taken down to a room. Just before that the police had ripped my Mac, but that's immaterial. I am trying to say this is the type of thing police do. They don't ask questions, their only concern is the children. I am telling you this because this is what must be happening to other people in the same situation.

When I was at the police station they thought I was going to be violent. When I was taken to Glenside, so two or three police came also. Obviously, they were very surprised when we got to the other end and I just got up and walked to the ward. They were very shocked so obviously they need training as well.

I go to a meeting now at Gloucester House and I would like some of the doctors or nurses to hear this. I would like to bring it to the next meeting, or one of the meetings to talk about it. I am more at ease when I am home on my own like this, talking into a tape than talking to a crowd of people. I am terribly interested in people, especially when they are going through a breakdown.

Something happened one morning in work. I am not going to say where I work. One of the staff had to go to someone's home. They were very perturbed as someone in the house was ill but didn't realise they were ill. They went round to the house and another member of the family was in a pickle, as they didn't know what action to take. They called in Social Services. This is what I am trying to cut out and why I'm trying to get a mobile telephone.

What does a person do if someone doesn't want to go to the doctor, or they do not feel they are ill? Does the parent or relation go to the doctor and get the doctor to call? I don't know because you are supposed to have the patient's permission, and that is a very tight thing. I don't know what my children are supposed to have done - they didn't do anything.

I did not realise at the time that I was ill and doing silly things, at home and at work. One thing I did was to buy a bottle of Bristol Milk, put it in a plastic container and each time I got to a desk and got depressed I would go out and have a drink from the container. The depression was coming very quick, one minute off, one minute on, one minute off.

My children thought I was becoming an alcoholic. I thought it was very funny but they didn't, anyway, I am trying to explain how it was that I felt.

In Glenside Hospital all patients in the hospital would benefit from having an animal in the hospital, such as a cat or dog. I think this would help greatly. It would help to calm them down a lot.

When people are in a state of illness because of nervous breakdown, and they want to call their doctor out, the doctor doesn't really want to come and see you. They tell you to have a nice cup of tea and a tablet and to go to bed. It is not so easy as that. What the patient needs is for the doctor to come and see them sit down and talk to them for a few minutes, and this would have a very calming effect on the patient. Perhaps someone from Gloucester House will be able to do this in the future, such as a nurse or doctor.

Just to have someone to talk to you for five minutes means much, much more than having another tablet.

Acknowledging a breakdown when someone does for instance can become very distressing. Ordinary people can't understand it. For the patient there seems to be no ending to it. On the way you think you have a friend but sometimes they are not your friend at all and you find out when you are in an illness. Some people when they go to work are in a breakdown, do silly things at work, like I have myself, their boss doesn't understand and take the 'mickey' out of them. They think that you cannot understand what they are saying. You try and get on with your work as well as possible, but it is not easy because when the person gets back to normal every so often they realise what people are saying, but they never understand what you are feeling.

All people suffering from a breakdown do lose their dignity because of being put down all the time. You want to yell at people and tell them not to be so stupid all the time. These people make you feel ten times worse than you are. We are told that when we are in a breakdown we are very odd and silly people. We are told to pull yourselves together and get on with it.

I'd like to see them pull themselves together if they were having a breakdown.

They are usually the type of people who would be begging others for help. But when you are in a deep, deep illness it shows anger, and anger can be terrible. Like I said you could go and smash a window.

I know of someone who gathered all their possessions in the middle of the room and nearly set fire to them. They were only stopped by their son coming in and stopping them. Some people are difficult, very difficult, and don't understand why they are doing these things. I am going by myself and other people suffering a breakdown. Some people sit in their chairs and do not want to get up, some work all the time, and you can work much faster in a breakdown, a hell of a lot faster. You do this to get the distress and anger out. One thing I did during my breakdown – I have a lot of bushes at the back of my house and I could get through cutting them in about twenty minutes. Normally it would take me a couple of hours.

Some people walk all the time and cry, they are just asking for help all the time – that's what they are trying to say. If people could learn about illness at school, the same as a history lesson or first aid lesson, they would have more of an idea what mental illness is like.

Perhaps they could be taught about mental illness as in the past when it was likened to the village idiot, and the progress that has been made since those days. If they were taught that mental illness is a sickness just like any other illness, then they might have a better appreciation of what someone in the throes of a breakdown are going through. Why can't teachers be taught about illness – they are taught about wars and everything else.

## Chapter 9

There is something else I want to say. When I was in my breakdown and I didn't know much about it at the time, I did not know much about tablets and their effects.

I used to think there were crowds of people outside coming after my friend, trying to chase my friend around the neighbourhood, but there was no one there at all. This was the effect of tablets. I know this now that I am back in the normal world. Some people see spiders and snakes climbing up the wall. I saw people and that was very, very frightening. I expect there are a lot of other people who would like to say a lot of things about the side effects of tablets. I tried to tell them at Glenside all the time, I think I mentioned this at the beginning, I used to try and tell people but they took no notice of me.

In time I told so many people that they had to take me into the office and sit me down. I was very scared at the time. I was trying to show them pieces of fluff on the floor – these little bits of fluff on the floor, and what they were doing at the time. This was not very easy for me because I was frightened. I expect a lot of people would like to try and turn around and tell people about these illusions, but a lot of people do not know when they are in a state of breakdown. I have had people say to me that's part of the breakdown, but no, it wasn't, not at all.

It's because of tablets you are given and their side effects. I don't think I can say much more about this, but if someone would like to talk on it, then they can.

The effects of the tablets makes them feel that they aren't really there. This is because they haven't been given a side effect tablet. I have had people say to me that that's part of the breakdown, but as I've said before, it isn't, and it's because no side effects tablet has been given.

When the children are very young and they have a very disturbed manner, this could have started from the time they are in the womb.

If you have a very disturbed person carrying a child, the body knows and the child knows that something is wrong. If it is a very disturbed person who is carrying the baby, the unborn baby can sense that disturbance. A few years after the baby is born it could become very naughty and unmanageable, and in years to come develop a breakdown. When asked about their past, that person could become very distressed.

That is why now a doctor will always ask questions about your background, because the mental illness could have stemmed from the disturbance the baby felt before it was even born. There could have been arguments in that house, all kinds of disturbances, and the poor child is going through it. When the child starts being naughty, it is told to shut up, go to school, and be quiet. Why can't the situation be dealt with then, while they are still innocent children, and not left until they are adults to develop a breakdown and get sent off to Barrow Gurney or Glenside.

When people are having tablets, any kind of tablets, and especially in breakdowns as I am doing, they should not smoke a cigarette just after taking a tablet. I have found that if you do, it gives you the impression that you are floating on air.

I tried this on myself many times. Tobacco is very strong and the stronger the tablets the worse it is. It is best to leave a time between taking the tablets and smoking a cigarette, it helps tremendously.

I should like to make some comments arising from my own experiences, and those of other people who have talked to me.

The attitude of some psychiatrists far from helping the patients actually hinders their recovery. Many patients are scared of authority and an arrogant manner, which talks down to them, does not encourage them to express what they are feeling and what their anxieties are.

They also apply labels to patients and henceforth continue to classify

them regardless of the fact that the original condition may no longer exist.

When help is really needed it is not available. It should be possible to have a quiet chat when a crisis situation arises. Instead, one first has to make an appointment with a GP and then a wait before seeing a consultant, by which time the urgency has passed. It is then not accepted that the problem has passed but one is still branded as having the problem.

It is worth mentioning that family or carers may, although they have the best of intentions, hinder recovery of a person who has suffered a breakdown. Instead of treating them normally and encouraging them to get on with their life, they continue to pamper them, being afraid that it may re-occur.

The beginning of life takes place in the womb. In a family where there is anger, distress or strife, these feelings communicate themselves to the unborn baby, whose mind can then become distorted or changed.

No evidence of this may be seen directly, possibly for years. At some time in their lives, sometimes triggered by a tragedy, but not always, may then develop stress symptoms.

They then go to the doctor who prescribes tablets or refers them to the hospital. Unfortunately, they cannot help the situation because it is due to what happened a long time ago in the womb and they do not know how to deal with it.

Sometimes they do not try to get help but endeavour to cope with the situation in their own way. This is rarely successful, although it may be where the original influence was not too severe.

What is really required is a building or room somewhere, which would be a drop-in centre. There, it would be possible to talk with other people in a similar situation, which would help to eradicate the feeling of isolation and helplessness. Also, there might be someone who could advise them if they thought medical attention was needed. This might well prevent the bizarre behaviour, which sometimes develops such as juggling with the traffic on a busy road.

Gladys Medcroft, December 1991.

End of tape recording.

Gladys Medcroft

**Chapter 10**

A crisis in one's life will often precipitate a breakdown. You are carrying on with life, people will ask you what is wrong. You know you are enduring pressure but are not sure what it is. You continue the daily routine of shopping and looking after the family.

The people you hurt the most are those closest to you, whoever they may be. They can't understand why, or the opposite you do nothing and they come home from work, tired, and find no cleaning done or no meal ready. All of a sudden you feel everyone is against you and you hit out at them. It takes a long time before you realise that you need to see a doctor. They normally give you tablets, say "take a rest … have a holiday." They do not see you early enough. All you are trying to do is hang on to life, if you can call it that; it is really existing without functioning.

Some people sit and do nothing all the time and shut themselves off. You try to talk to them but they cannot realise that other people have been through the same experience.

You try and tell them there is a light at the end of the tunnel, but there is no convincing them. The opposite, which I experienced, is over activity; I worked day and night, and this therapy helped me through the crisis. You can never relax in comfort, always being alert and ready to pounce on someone; always waiting for something to happen, but it never does, especially if someone is trying to help you.

If you are trying to help someone, maybe at first there is no response and they are very suspicious. But often they will return to you, and although they may not be ready to accept what you say, they are ready to trust you, which is a first step forward.

The worst time is at night when your imagination runs away with you. This may be aggravated in some cases by medication. Objects appear to be alive as a friend, which is safe and will not hurt you or let you down.

Some people go for long walks or bus rides, escaping from their own reality into another world, forgetting all responsibilities such as young children left in the house alone.

This may lead to dangerous complications such as the children being put into care. Other effects may involve talking in riddles, which people can't understand; one's concentration goes and the mind flits from one subject to another in rapid succession.

This may result in one losing one's job; while in this state the patient always thinks they are right regardless, and obviously this cannot be accepted where work is involved and might even be dangerous if the work is concerned with operating machinery.

There has been a small improvement in the general attitude to somewhat bizarre behaviour, which a person may be showing. Years ago, the only course of action was to call the police who, because you were acting abnormally and unable to explain why, took you off to the police station. There, some treated you like a criminal or quickly dispatched you to a mental hospital where you stayed for a long period.

Nowadays, a care officer could be contacted and a more humane approach would be adopted.

When you are getting insufficient sleep you get overtired, and although you may be desperately weary you have to get up and busy yourself doing housework, ironing, washing the floor etc. Even when you are asleep the brain is still in action, and you are suddenly awoken by what seems like an explosion in the head, which feels on all sides as if it is going to burst, and you want to scream. No one can explain to a doctor the feeling of a band around the head and the brain seems to be going faster and faster.

Since you cannot sleep at night you feel tired during the day and fall asleep at any odd time.

Give time to listen to a patient. They may not be able to talk right away and what they say may not make sense to the listener, but to the patient it will be true facts. It may not sound like the truth, but they believe it to be so and it is important not to walk away from them or indicate in any way that you do not believe them.

They need a friend and someone to be open minded.

The worst thing that can happen is that they feel rejected or disbelieved. At the same time do not push the patient for information as this may cause them to retreat within themselves and say nothing. When there is a physical defect such as a broken leg, treatment is obvious but in mental illness where there is no visible sign it is much more difficult.

When a patient is in hospital they should be allowed to behave as naturally as possible.

That is the way they would if they were at home. For example, if they want to get up in the night and make a cup of tea, this could be a first step towards independence.

In the same way let them prepare their own breakfast, even if it is just cereal and toast. Not everyone will want this facility, but it should be there for those who do. A visiting room should be provided and be a friendly place so that visitors can feel at home, where they can make a cup of tea and have a smoke and create a family atmosphere. This helps to rehabilitate the patient because it develops a natural environment. One serious problem after discharge is the loss of confidence. This is aggravated by others, who due to embarrassment of lack of understanding, cannot easily communicate with the patient and because of this they tend to ignore the person.

When one is in a breakdown there may be signs of violent behaviour, e.g. throwing a chair across the room.

This is revealed when some force outside the control of the person takes over and the person can do nothing to prevent it. It may last for just a few minutes or a lot longer. The behavioural pattern may not necessarily involve violence but always-bizarre unnatural behaviour, maybe dressing up, travelling in buses without any intention of going anywhere, setting fire to things. It is as if someone was ordering you to do these things.

It is important to make a distinction between a breakdown and mental illness. The former may be caused by various external circumstances such as a death in the family or social or financial deprivation. But the causes of mental illness are much more complicated and difficult to define.

This is partly due to the fact that behavioural patterns vary so much. For example, a person may be in a deep state of depression and totally withdrawn, but five minutes later or maybe a longer period they emerge from that state and be completely 'normal.' This could give a false impression, as a doctor might consider the patient being of a fit state to be discharged, when in actual fact their changed condition may be only temporary and a relapse may occur. Again, a patient in a depression may appear not to be noticing what is going on and not to be listening to what is being said, but in actual fact they are absorbing it all and can recollect it later.

On the main side effects of prolonged therapy with anti-depressants is worry and fear, which occur at intervals for no very obvious reason. This may lead to a compulsion to take extra medication, which will only make the situation worse.

The inner mind can play tricks on the body producing thoughts and actions, which are out of character and purposeless.

You know all the time what you want to do, but the mind tells you to do something different.

When seeing people or hearing voices give the mind something else to think about. One way to change the pattern is to give a loud shout from the stomach.

In some cases people are very uncaring and hurtful because they do not understand what mental illness is. They assume it means unintelligent or even simple mindedness, which is far from being the case. They are, in fact, no different from other people. If there is a dispute between two people one of whom has mental illness, the arbitrator will instinctively accept the word of the non-ill person, without considering the facts. This can make the ill person very angry.

The onset of a breakdown is a gradual process, during which the person concerned is aware that something unusual is happening, but other people don't recognise the changed pattern of behaviour.

It may take various forms but often the first indication is that people appear different.

These are frequently those one knows well, but may seem to be strangers. At the same time some part of the brain is functioning normally and, for example, one may say "sorry, I didn't recognise you, I haven't got my glasses on."

After a while behaviour may become more bizarre, manifested by strange uncharacteristic actions and thoughts. One may fear that someone is following them when no one is there. They may find themselves in the middle of the road directing the traffic, or talk to the clock on the oven or the characters on the TV screen. All the time some part of their mind can tell them that they are behaving irrationally.

A time comes when one feels that help is needed, so one goes to their GP. However, because of fear of being laughed at and ridiculed, much of the happenings, of which the above are examples, remain unsaid.

This may not be true in all cases, but in a large number I feel it is so. Usually medication is given, but if no improvement occurs and it usually doesn't although it may calm one down, a referral is made to a psychiatrist, or if necessary admission to hospital.

This is where the breakdown in treatment really occurs. On being faced by a psychiatrist, although a small percentage of patients will talk, most will not.

The vast majority takes refuge in silence, they do not want to be labelled. This is particularly true in subsequent breakdowns. Also there is the fear that the more you reveal the longer will be the stay in hospital, which seems like a prison sentence.

Instead of interrogation, I feel there should be more group therapy among the patients and ex-patients. Also more occupational and physiotherapy would help those in need.

Gladys Medcroft

## Chapter 11

Some years went by and I thought all my problems were behind me, but one can never be completely free from the fear that fate has another blow in store. Suddenly, due to a crisis situation, things changed, and I developed phobias.

The initial one was a fear of traffic and travelling, both on public and private transport. On one occasion, while on holiday at Dawlish, we had booked to go by coach to a show in Torquay.

The driver chose to avoid the main route as he said the other road was more scenic. It was also very bumpy and a longer journey so he had to drive fast. I was terrified and wanted to get off, but although I was screaming, no one took any notice. Eventually we arrived. I was too frightened to enjoy the show – Cannon and Ball – as I was worried as to how I was going to get back, but I told a couple sitting in front of me that we shouldn't be on the coach. It resulted in having to get a taxi back and I wouldn't let the driver go faster than 40 mph.

Strangely enough train travel did not give me any problems. Looking back, I think my fear of cars, coaches etc., might stem from the time when my husband was so ill and suffering frequent blackouts, but still insisted on driving the car.

It caused a great problem in my life as I was afraid to go anywhere, and I couldn't see how it could be resolved. However, I was introduced to relaxation exercises, and as a result of exercising every day, I can now travel on buses by myself.

If I feel myself getting tense, I quietly do some breathing exercises, which relax me.

Then there were dogs to make my life a misery. In the district where I live there are a lot of stray dogs. One particular day, four of these dogs rushed at me. I don't know if they intended to attack or if they were roaming in a pack, but to me they represented a ferocious menace.

Fortunately, I had my shopping trolley with me, which I used to protect myself, and meantime a man drove them off. After that I was unable to go out alone. I saw dogs when there were none there. My son and daughter went with me whenever possible and their arms were black and blue where I grabbed them whenever I saw a dog, even if it was a long way off.

To get to work, which really wasn't very far, was a nightmare. I would attach myself to anyone who was about, or run inside gateways. I couldn't even endure seeing a dog on television. I knew I must get treatment and took the necessary steps, involving attending hospital as a day patient. At first I looked at pictures of dogs in books, particularly Alsatians, which represented the greatest danger to me.

The next step was to find a docile dog I could get familiar with. A lady who lives quite near and has such a dog, kindly agreed that I might call on her and this I did, accompanied by one of the doctors. It took quite a few visits. At first, I could only speak to the dog from a distance, but eventually I progressed to stroking him but only in the presence of the owner and doctor. I don't think I could have done it if I had been there alone.

Having mastered this step I was taken to another house where an Alsatian lived. This was a very different proposition. I think it was the size of the animal that made the difference, and was a slow progress.

First the dog was put in the garden with the window slightly open. Toby, as he was called, could just put his nose in the gap and I eventually managed to stroke it. The next stage was for the door to be held slightly ajar and I would stroke his head. I continued like this for a few weeks. Then the owner would put Toby on the lead in the garden and I had to walk past and try and smooth him as I went. I knew in my heart it was perfectly safe but I still found it frightening. It was quite a little journey to this house and if on the way he saw a group of dogs, the doctor would stop the car and encourage me to walk past them.

To go back to Toby. The lead was taken off him and I found my confidence improved gradually until I lost my fear of him and could approach and smooth him, without a sense of horror. Happily, now I have thanks to the treatment I received, overcome my fear of dogs.

I have found great assistance from practising relaxation exercises. At first I did these to the accompaniment of a tape but no longer need this, and I have been able to lend it to others who have also derived benefit from the exercises.

I am now thankfully in control of my actions and able to go out on my own and live my life to the full.

## Chapter 12

If you have been trying to trace, without success, a member of your family whom you haven't seen for many years, or perhaps never, don't be discouraged but keep following up any avenues, which may be helpful.

I have previously written about my childhood and explained how all the children were brought up separately. I had not seen my youngest brother for nearly thirty years, when he was eight years old. I followed up various channels – writing to the papers, contacting the children's department etc.

Eventually a Social Services worker, Mary Rowe was successful in tracing him to Birmingham. He came to visit and it was a highly emotional meeting, especially as looking at him I could see a replica of myself.

Since our first meeting we have remained in touch and I have had the pleasure of meeting his family.

My older brother John, I briefly met when my children were small, but due to the fact that he lost his memory and I didn't have his address, I lost contact. However, recently the local paper printed a piece for me regarding my search, which was happily seen by his solicitor, who rang me and subsequently we have re-united.

So do not be discouraged if you are in such a situation and you may have much pleasure in store.

**Chapter 13**

When one is suffering from a mental illness, there may be many different aspects and one of the strangest phenomena is the interpretation of body movements and their reaction to them.

I will give you some examples as they have been told to me: -

"When someone looked at the ceiling, I thought there was someone there, telling me to go away."

"If my slippers were facing the wrong way, or if my wardrobe was open with the clothes visible, they were giving me a message, which I did not always understand, sometimes frightening and sometimes not."

"If someone is tapping their foot or any other part of the body, they are telling me to go away."

"It's like the good people were telling the bad people about me, and if I was on the bus stop they could be saying that you must go away."

That is typical of some of the thoughts that go through your mind.

One of the problems caused by medication used in cases of mental illness is the side effects caused. Among these, weight changes produce a real worry. In some cases there is a weight loss, but much more frequently there is a substantial weight gain. This can cause a loss of self-respect. The patients are often those least able to replenish their wardrobe as required. Consequently they wear clothes which no longer fit them and lose interest in their appearance. I feel a grant in these circumstances would be more than justified.

Struggling in stony soil,

Battling against wind and rain,

The red rose blossoms

Giving its message of hope and love,

But soon, alas, its frail petals fade and die,

Warmed by the sun,

Cared for by gentle hands,

It thrives and endures.

So with the body,

Starved of affection, warmth and love,

The mind shrivels and dies,

Give me your love and strength,

To feed my soul,

Without it I am dead.

G. Medcroft.